SOMATIC EXERCISES FOR SENIORS

10 Minutes Daily Exercises To Improve Flexibility, Mobility And Reduce Belly Fat Quickly With 50 Day Plan

DR. PERSIS HILLARY

TABLE OF CONTENTS

INTRODUCTION

SOMATIC YOGA FOR SENIORS

HOW TO USE THIS GUIDE

Certainly, here's a list of 40 somatic exercises suitable for seniors:

1. Neck Tilts

2. Shoulder Rolls

3. Arm Circles

4. Wrist Flexion and Extension

5. Ankle Rolls

6. Seated Marching

7. Gentle Spine Twists

8. Pelvic Tilts

9. Cat-Cow Stretch

10. Knee-to-Chest Stretch

11. Seated Leg Extensions

12. Ankle Flex and Point

13. Seated Side Bends

14. Hip Circles

15. Toe Taps

16. Heel Slides

17. Butterfly Stretch

18. Chest Openers

19. Upper Back Stretch

20. Seated Forward Bend

21. Elbow Circles

22. Chin Tucks

23. Leg Swings

24. Torso Circles

25. Finger Stretches

26. Gentle Squats

27. Seated Torso Twists

28. Standing Hip Flexor Stretch

29. Calf Raises

30. Hamstring Stretch

31. Wrist Circles

32. Shoulder Blade Squeeze

33. Standing Side Stretch

34. Seated Knee Lifts

35. Clamshells

36. Bird Dog Stretch

37. Seated Hamstring Stretch

38. Wall Push-Ups

39. Balance Exercises (like one-leg stands)

40. Deep Diaphragmatic Breathing

50 DAY EXERCISE PLAN FOR SENIORS

INTRODUCTION

Somatic exercises, a form of movement therapy, are increasingly recognized as an effective way to enhance the well-being of seniors. These exercises focus on internal physical perception and experience, offering a gentle approach to movement that emphasizes bodily awareness and mindfulness. As individuals age, maintaining physical health and mobility becomes crucial. Somatic exercises provide a means to not only sustain but also improve flexibility, strength, and coordination in a manner that is respectful of the body's limits and capabilities.

Unlike more strenuous forms of exercise, somatic practices are centered around gentle, controlled movements that help in reconnecting with the body and understanding its signals. This mindful approach to movement aids in reducing stress, easing chronic pain, and improving posture, which are common concerns among the elderly population. Additionally, these exercises can be easily modified to suit individual needs and abilities, making them accessible to seniors with varying levels of physical fitness.

Furthermore, practicing somatic exercises regularly can lead to increased body awareness. This heightened awareness is instrumental in preventing falls and injuries, common concerns in senior care. By integrating these exercises into their daily routine, seniors can enjoy an improved quality of life, with greater independence and a stronger connection to their bodies.

SOMATIC YOGA FOR SENIORS

Somatic Yoga for Seniors

Somatic Yoga, a practice that emphasizes internal physical perception and experience, holds significant benefits for seniors. This gentle form of yoga focuses on the somatic exercises that encourage body awareness, flexibility, and relaxation, tailored specifically for older adults.

Key Aspects of Somatic Yoga for Seniors

1. Mind-Body Connection: Somatic Yoga fosters a deep connection between the mind and body. By concentrating on internal sensations and movements, seniors can enhance their body awareness, leading to improved balance and coordination.

2. Gentle Movements: Unlike traditional yoga, Somatic Yoga for seniors involves slow, gentle movements that are ideal for older bodies. These movements help in maintaining flexibility, reducing muscle stiffness, and increasing range of motion.

3. Stress Reduction: The practice includes deep breathing and mindfulness techniques, which are excellent for reducing stress and anxiety, common issues among seniors.

4. Pain Management: Regular practice can lead to a decrease in chronic pain, a common concern for many seniors, by releasing tension and improving muscle function.

5. Improved Posture and Balance: Somatic Yoga strengthens core muscles, which are essential for good posture and balance, reducing the risk of falls.

Sample Exercises in Somatic Yoga for Seniors

1. Pelvic Tilts: Lying on the back, gently arching and flattening the lower back. This movement enhances lower back flexibility and awareness.

2. Cat-Cow Stretch: On all fours, alternately arching and rounding the spine. This exercise increases spine flexibility.

3. Seated Twists: Gentle spinal twists while seated, focusing on the sensation of movement in the spine.

4. Shoulder Lifts and Drops: Raising and lowering the shoulders to relieve tension in the shoulder and neck area.

5. Leg Extensions: While seated or lying down, gently extending each leg to strengthen the thigh muscles and improve joint health.

6. Ankle Rolls and Flexes: Rotating and flexing the ankles, which helps in maintaining ankle flexibility and reducing stiffness.

7. Diaphragmatic Breathing: Focusing on deep, abdominal breathing to enhance lung capacity and promote relaxation.

Conclusion

Somatic Yoga for seniors is an accessible and beneficial way to maintain physical health and mental well-being. By focusing on the internal experience of movement, seniors can achieve a greater sense of body awareness and control. This practice not only improves physical attributes like balance, flexibility, and strength but also contributes to emotional and psychological health through stress reduction and mindfulness. Regular practice can lead to a significant enhancement of the overall quality of life for seniors.

HOW TO USE THIS GUIDE

How to Use This Guide for Somatic Exercises for Seniors

Welcome to Your Journey of Movement and Wellness

This guide is designed to help seniors engage in somatic exercises safely and effectively. Somatic exercises are gentle, mindful movements that focus on internal perception and experience. They are particularly beneficial for seniors, as they enhance body awareness, improve flexibility, and reduce stress. Here's how to make the most of this guide:

1. Start Slowly: If you're new to somatic exercises, begin with shorter sessions. Gradually increase the duration as you become more comfortable.

2. Choose a Comfortable Space: Ensure you have a quiet, spacious area to perform these exercises. A flat, non-slippery surface is ideal.

3. Listen to Your Body: Somatic exercises are all about internal awareness. Pay close attention to how your body feels during each movement. If something hurts or feels uncomfortable, stop and adjust.

4. Consistency is Key: Regular practice yields the best results. Aim to incorporate these exercises into your daily routine.

5. Focus on Breathing: Proper breathing is a central part of somatic exercises. Inhale and exhale deeply and slowly through your nose, synchronizing your breath with your movements.

6. Use Props if Needed: Feel free to use chairs, cushions, or walls for support, especially for balance and stability exercises.

7. Stay Hydrated: Drink water before and after your exercise session to keep your body well-hydrated.

8. Wear Appropriate Clothing: Comfortable, loose-fitting clothing allows for unrestricted movement.

9. Mix and Match: Feel free to combine different exercises from this guide. Tailor your routine to suit your preferences and physical needs.

10. Seek Professional Advice: If you have any health concerns or if you're recovering from an injury, consult with a healthcare professional before starting these exercises.

11. Enjoy the Process: Remember, the goal is to enhance your body awareness and overall wellbeing. Enjoy the process and the gentle journey of exploring your body's capabilities.

12. Track Your Progress: Keep a simple record of your daily practice. Note any changes in your flexibility, balance, and overall wellbeing.

13. Stay Patient and Positive: Progress may be gradual, but with regular practice, you will notice improvements in your body's function and your general health.

Remember, somatic exercises are not just physical movements; they are a pathway to better understand and care for your body. Enjoy this journey of gentle exploration and self-care.

SOMATIC EXERCISES FOR SENIORS

Certainly! Here are step-by-step instructions for performing each of these somatic exercises, tailored for seniors:

1. Neck Tilts

1. Position: Sit comfortably in a chair with your back straight and feet flat on the floor.

2. Relax: Start by relaxing your shoulders and gently resting your hands on your lap.

3. Tilt Downward: Slowly tilt your head forward, aiming to bring your chin towards your chest. Hold this position for a few seconds.

4. Return to Center: Gently lift your head back to the starting position.

5. Side Tilts: Now, gently tilt your head to the right, bringing your ear towards the shoulder. Hold, then return to the center. Repeat on the left side.

6. Repeat: Do this sequence a few times, ensuring smooth and slow movements.

2. Shoulder Rolls

1. Position: Sit or stand with your back straight.

2. Roll Forward: Lift your shoulders up towards your ears, then roll them forward, down, and then back, creating a circular motion.

3. Reverse Direction: After several forward rolls, reverse the direction, rolling your shoulders backward, up, forward, and down.

4. Repeat: Do around 5 rolls in each direction.

3. Arm Circles

1. Position: Stand with your feet shoulder-width apart. Extend your arms out to the sides at shoulder height.

2. Circle Forward: Slowly make small circles with your arms, moving forward. Start with small circles, gradually making them larger.

3. Reverse Direction: After about 10 circles, switch directions and circle your arms backward.

4. Repeat: Do 10 circles in each direction.

4. Wrist Flexion and Extension

1. Position: Sit or stand comfortably. Extend one arm forward, palm facing down.

2. Flexion: Gently bend your wrist to point your fingers towards the floor. Hold for a few seconds.

3. Extension: Then, gently bend your wrist to point your fingers upwards. Hold for a few seconds.

4. Switch Hands: Repeat the same movements with the other hand.

5. Repeat: Do 5-10 repetitions with each hand.

5. Ankle Rolls

1. Position: Sit in a chair with your feet flat on the ground.

2. Lift One Foot: Lift one foot off the ground, keeping your leg bent at the knee.

3. Roll Ankle: Slowly roll your ankle in a circular motion. Start with small circles, then gradually increase the size.

4. Reverse Direction: After several circles, switch directions.

5. Switch Feet: Repeat the exercise with the other foot.

6. Repeat: Do 5-10 circles in each direction with each ankle.

Certainly! Here are step-by-step instructions for performing the listed somatic exercises. These exercises are gentle and can be beneficial for seniors, focusing on improving flexibility, balance, and body awareness.

1. Seated Marching

Objective: To improve lower body strength and coordination.

Steps:

1. Sit on a sturdy chair with your back straight and feet flat on the floor.

2. Lift your right knee towards your chest as high as comfortable, then lower it back to the starting position.

3. Repeat with your left knee.

4. Continue alternating legs, mimicking a marching motion.

5. Perform this exercise for 1-2 minutes, maintaining a steady, controlled pace.

 2. Gentle Spine Twists

Objective: To enhance spinal mobility and flexibility.

Steps:

1. Sit upright in a chair with your feet flat on the ground.

2. Place your left hand on your right knee and your right hand behind you on the seat of the chair.

3. Gently twist your torso to the right, looking over your right shoulder. Hold for a few seconds.

4. Return to the center and repeat on the other side, placing your right hand on your left knee and your left hand behind you.

5. Perform 5-10 twists on each side, moving slowly and smoothly.

3. Pelvic Tilts

Objective: To strengthen the lower back and improve pelvic mobility.

Steps:

1. Sit on the edge of a chair with your feet flat on the floor and hands on your hips.

2. Gently arch your lower back and stick out your buttocks, tilting your pelvis forward.

3. Hold for a few seconds, then slowly tilt your pelvis backward, rounding your lower back.

4. Move back and forth between these positions smoothly.

5. Repeat this motion 10-15 times.

4. Cat-Cow Stretch

Objective: To increase spine flexibility and relieve tension in the back.

Steps:

1. Start on your hands and knees on a comfortable surface, with your wrists under your shoulders and knees under your hips.

2. Inhale and arch your back, tilting your tailbone and chin upward (Cow Pose).

3. Exhale and round your spine, tucking your chin to your chest and drawing your belly button toward your spine (Cat Pose).

4. Continue this sequence for 1-2 minutes, flowing smoothly between Cat and Cow poses.

5. Knee-to-Chest Stretch

Objective: To stretch the lower back and hips.

Steps:

1. Lie on your back on a comfortable surface, with your legs extended and arms at your sides.

2. Bend your right knee and bring it towards your chest, clasping your hands around your shin.

3. Hold the stretch for 15-30 seconds, feeling a gentle pull in your lower back and hip.

4. Slowly release and repeat with your left leg.

5. Alternate legs for 5-10 repetitions each.

Remember to breathe deeply and steadily during these exercises. If you feel any pain or discomfort, stop immediately and consult with a healthcare professional. Regular practice can lead to improvements in flexibility, balance, and overall well-being.

Certainly! Here are step-by-step instructions for each of the listed somatic exercises, tailored for seniors:

11. Seated Leg Extensions

1. Start Position: Sit in a sturdy chair with your feet flat on the floor and your back straight. Hold onto the sides of the chair for support.

2. Extend One Leg: Slowly extend one leg out in front of you, keeping your foot flexed (toes pointing upwards).

3. Return to Start: Lower the leg back to the starting position. Keep the movement controlled and smooth.

4. Alternate Legs: Repeat the movement with the other leg.

5. Repetitions: Do 8-10 repetitions for each leg.

12. Ankle Flex and Point

1. Start Position: Sit comfortably with your legs extended in front of you. You can do this either sitting on the floor, on a bed, or in a chair.

2. Flex Your Ankle: Slowly flex your ankle by pulling your toes up towards you.

3. Point Your Toes: Then, gently point your toes away from you, stretching the front of the ankle.

4. Repetitions: Repeat this flex and point movement 10-15 times.

13. Seated Side Bends

1. Start Position: Sit in a chair with your feet flat on the floor, spine straight, and arms at your sides.

2. Side Bend: Raise one arm overhead and gently bend your torso to the opposite side. Keep your other hand on your thigh or the side of the chair for support.

3. Return to Center: Slowly come back to the starting position.

4. Alternate Sides: Repeat on the other side.

5. Repetitions: Do 5-8 bends on each side.

14. Hip Circles

1. Start Position: Stand behind a chair or next to a support for balance, feet hip-width apart.

2. Circle Your Hip: Lift one leg and make small circles with the hip. Keep your standing leg slightly bent for stability.

3. Change Directions: After 5-10 circles, switch directions.

4. Alternate Legs: Repeat with the other leg.

5. Repetitions: Do 5-10 circles in each direction for each leg.

15. Toe Taps

1. Start Position: Sit in a chair with your feet flat on the floor.

2. Tap Your Toes: Lift the toes of one foot while keeping your heel on the ground, and then tap your toes back down.

3. Alternate Feet: Repeat with the other foot.

4. Repetitions: Do 10-15 taps with each foot.

Certainly! Here are step-by-step instructions for each of the specified somatic exercises:

16. Heel Slides

1. Lie on your back on a comfortable, flat surface.

2. Bend your knees, keeping your feet flat on the ground.

3. Slowly straighten one leg, sliding your heel along the ground.

4. Slide your heel back, returning to the starting position.

5. Repeat 10 times with one leg, then switch to the other leg.

17. Butterfly Stretch

1. Sit on the floor with your back straight.

2. Bring the soles of your feet together in front of you.

3. Gently press your knees towards the floor using your elbows or hands.

4. Hold the stretch for 20-30 seconds, breathing deeply.

5. Release and repeat 2-3 times.

18. Chest Openers

1. Stand or sit with your back straight.

2. Clasp your hands behind your back.

3. Gently lift your arms up and away from your body, opening your chest.

4. Hold for 15-20 seconds while breathing deeply.

5. Relax and repeat 2-3 times.

19. Upper Back Stretch

1. Sit or stand with your back straight.

2. Extend your arms in front of you and clasp your hands together.

3. Round your upper back, pushing your clasped hands away from you.

4. Lower your head slightly, feeling the stretch in your upper back.

5. Hold for 20-30 seconds, then relax.

6. Repeat 2-3 times.

20. Seated Forward Bend

1. Sit on the floor with your legs extended in front of you.

2. Inhale and extend your arms overhead.

3. Exhale and bend forward from your hips, reaching towards your toes.

4. Hold the position for 20-30 seconds, breathing deeply.

5. Slowly rise back to the seated position.

6. Repeat 2-3 times.

21. Elbow Circles

1. Stand or sit with your back straight.

2. Bend your elbows and touch your shoulders with your fingertips.

3. Circle your elbows in a forward motion 5-10 times.

4. Reverse the motion, circling backward 5-10 times.

22. Chin Tucks

1. Sit or stand with your spine straight.

2. Gently pull your chin back, creating a "double chin."

3. Hold for 5 seconds.

4. Release and return to the starting position.

5. Repeat 10 times.

23. Leg Swings

1. Stand next to a wall or chair for support.

2. Shift your weight to one leg.

3. Gently swing the other leg forward and backward.

4. Perform 10 swings, then switch to the other leg.

5. For side leg swings, swing your leg left and right across your body, 10 times on each leg.

Certainly! Here are step-by-step instructions for each of the somatic exercises listed:

24. Torso Circles:

1. Stand with your feet shoulder-width apart, knees slightly bent.

2. Place your hands on your hips.

3. Slowly begin to move your torso in a circular motion.

4. Keep your movements smooth and controlled.

5. Circle five times in one direction, then switch and circle five times in the other direction.

25. Finger Stretches:

1. Extend your arms in front of you at shoulder height.

2. Spread your fingers wide apart, then close them into a fist.

3. Repeat this opening and closing motion slowly 10 times.

4. Then, gently bend each finger individually for a deeper stretch.

26. Gentle Squats:

1. Stand with feet hip-width apart.

2. Extend your arms in front of you for balance.

3. Bend your knees, lowering your body as if sitting back into a chair.

4. Keep your back straight and avoid extending your knees past your toes.

5. Lower down as far as comfortable, then slowly stand back up.

6. Perform 8-10 squats, as long as it feels comfortable.

27. Seated Torso Twists:

1. Sit in a chair with your feet flat on the floor.

2. Keep your spine tall and shoulders relaxed.

3. Place your right hand on your left knee and your left hand behind you for support.

4. Gently twist your torso to the left, looking over your left shoulder.

5. Hold for a few breaths, then return to the center.

6. Repeat on the opposite side.

28. Standing Hip Flexor Stretch:

1. Stand up straight and take a step back with your right foot.

2. Bend your left knee, keeping your right leg straight behind you.

3. Lean forward slightly, keeping your back straight.

4. Hold the stretch for 15-30 seconds.

5. Repeat with the left leg stepped back.

29. Calf Raises:

1. Stand upright with your feet hip-width apart.

2. Raise up onto the balls of your feet, lifting your heels off the ground.

3. Hold the position for a second at the top.

4. Slowly lower your heels back to the ground.

5. Repeat this motion for 10-15 raises.

30. Hamstring Stretch:

1. Sit on the floor with one leg extended and the other bent, foot against the inner thigh.

2. Lean forward from your hips towards your extended foot.

3. Reach for your toes or ankle, depending on your flexibility.

4. Hold for 15-30 seconds.

5. Switch legs and repeat.

31. Wrist Circles:

1. Extend your arms in front of you with palms facing down.

2. Slowly rotate your wrists in a circular motion.

3. Do 10 circles in one direction, then switch to 10 circles in the opposite direction.

32. Shoulder Blade Squeeze:

1. Sit or stand with your back straight.

2. Imagine you are holding a pencil between your shoulder blades.

3. Squeeze your shoulder blades together, holding the 'pencil' in place.

4. Hold for 5 seconds, then release.

5. Repeat 10 times.

Certainly! Here are step-by-step instructions for performing each of these somatic exercises:

33. Standing Side Stretch

1. Stand with your feet hip-width apart, ensuring good balance.

2. Raise your right arm overhead and reach towards the left side, creating a gentle stretch along your right side.

3. Keep your left hand on your hip or let it hang by your side.

4. Hold the stretch for 15-30 seconds, breathing deeply.

5. Slowly return to the starting position and repeat on the other side.

34. Seated Knee Lifts

1. Sit in a sturdy chair without armrests, feet flat on the floor.

2. Engage your abdominal muscles gently.

3. Slowly lift your right knee towards your chest as far as comfortable.

4. Hold for a few seconds, then lower your foot back to the floor.

5. Repeat with the left leg. Alternate legs for 10-15 repetitions.

35. Clamshells

1. Lie on your side with legs stacked and knees bent at a 45-degree angle.

2. Rest your head on your lower arm, and use your other hand for stability.

3. Keeping your feet together, raise your upper knee as high as you can without shifting your hips.

4. Hold for a moment, then slowly lower the knee back down.

5. Perform 10-15 repetitions, then switch sides.

36. Bird Dog Stretch

1. Begin on your hands and knees with a flat back, hands under shoulders, knees under hips.

2. Extend your right arm forward and your left leg back, keeping both parallel to the floor.

3. Hold the position for a few seconds, then return to the starting position.

4. Repeat with the opposite arm and leg. Perform 10-15 repetitions on each side.

37. Seated Hamstring Stretch

1. Sit on the edge of a chair with one leg extended forward and the other bent.

2. Keep your back straight and lean forward gently from your hips towards the extended leg.

3. Reach towards your toes or shins, feeling a stretch in the back of your thigh.

4. Hold for 15-30 seconds, then switch legs and repeat.

38. Wall Push-Ups

1. Stand an arm's length away from a wall, feet shoulder-width apart.

2. Place your palms flat against the wall at shoulder height.

3. Bend your elbows to slowly bring your body towards the wall.

4. Push back to the starting position. Repeat for 10-15 repetitions.

39. Balance Exercises (One-Leg Stands)

1. Stand next to a chair or a wall for support.

2. Shift your weight onto one leg.

3. Slowly lift the other leg off the ground, holding it in the air for as long as you can maintain balance.

4. Lower the leg and repeat on the other side. Aim to hold each stand for 10-30 seconds.

40. Deep Diaphragmatic Breathing

1. Sit or lie comfortably, with one hand on your chest and the other on your abdomen.

2. Breathe in deeply through your nose, feeling your abdomen rise more than your chest.

3. Exhale slowly through your mouth, feeling the abdomen lower.

4. Repeat this deep breathing pattern for 3-5 minutes, focusing on the rise and fall of your abdomen.

Creating a 50-day exercise plan for seniors using the given somatic exercises involves a gradual progression that allows for rest and recovery. Each exercise can be adapted to individual fitness levels and any specific health concerns should be considered. Here's a suggested plan:

Weekly Structure:

- Day 1: Lower Body Focus

- Day 2: Upper Body Focus

- Day 3: Balance and Core

- Day 4: Rest or Gentle Walking

- Day 5: Full Body Stretch

- Day 6: Strength and Flexibility

- Day 7: Rest or Gentle Walking

Daily Breakdown (repeat each week for 50 days):

Day 1 - Lower Body Focus

- Seated Knee Lifts: 10-15 reps each leg

- Clamshells: 10-15 reps each side

- Seated Hamstring Stretch: Hold for 15-30 seconds each leg

Day 2 - Upper Body Focus

- Wall Push-Ups: 10-15 reps

- Arm Circles: 10 reps in each direction

- Shoulder Rolls: 10 reps

Day 3 - Balance and Core

- Balance Exercises (One-Leg Stands): Hold each stand for 10-30 seconds

- Bird Dog Stretch: 10-15 reps each side

- Deep Diaphragmatic Breathing: 3-5 minutes

Day 4 - Rest or Gentle Walking

- Engage in light activities like walking, gardening, or gentle yoga

- Focus on maintaining activity levels without strain

Day 5 - Full Body Stretch

- Standing Side Stretch: Hold for 15-30 seconds each side

- Gentle Spine Twists: 10 reps each side

- Butterfly Stretch: Hold for 15-30 seconds

Day 6 - Strength and Flexibility

- Repeat a combination of exercises from Day 1, Day 2, and Day 3 but at a lower intensity or fewer reps

Day 7 - Rest or Gentle Walking

- Similar to Day 4, focus on light, enjoyable activities that keep you moving without exertion

Notes:

1. Adaptation: Adjust the number of repetitions and duration of stretches according to your comfort level.

2. Progression: As you advance, gradually increase repetitions or stretching duration.

3. Hydration: Drink water before and after workouts.

4. Warm-Up and Cool-Down: Start each session with a 5-minute warm-up (like walking in place) and end with a 5-minute cool-down.

5. Listen to Your Body: If an exercise causes pain or discomfort, stop doing it and consult a healthcare professional.

6. Enjoy the Process: The goal is to maintain mobility, flexibility, and strength, so make sure to enjoy your exercise routine!

Remember, regularity and consistency are more important than intensity in a senior exercise program. It's about maintaining overall health and well-being.